How To Help Eliminate Low Back Pain And Achieve Long Term Relief

Your All In One Guide To Understanding Lower Back Pain And Preventing A Relapse

LOUISE HAMPTON

How to Help Eliminate Low Back Pain and Achieve Long Term Relief

Copyright © 2018 Louise Hampton
ISBN: 978-1-912243-44-0

Published by
The Endless Bookcase Ltd

71 Castle Road, St Albans, Hertfordshire, England UK, AL1 5DQ

All rights reserved.

This book is not intended as a substitute for the medical advice of physicians. The reader should regularly consult a physician in matters relating to his/her health and particularly with respect to any symptoms that may require diagnosis or medical attention.

Printed Edition

This book is available in a variety of formats both paper and electronic.

ACKNOWLEDGEMENTS

A big thank you to my husband for all his help and support with this book. I could not have done it without him. Thank you to my mum, dad and family for their support over the years. Thank you to my good friend Sarah Townsend for looking through the book from a chiropractic point of view, to my mother-in-law Wendy Hampton for proof reading and to Catherine Quinn the President of the British Chiropractic Association, for her input. Thank you to Landmark Editorial and The Endless Bookcase for their help, and to Pret-a-Portrait and Shot by Hobbs for all the photographs in the book. I dedicate this book to my wonderful children Toby and Zara.

ABOUT THE AUTHOR

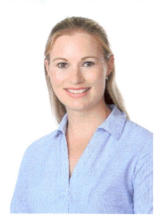

Dr Louise Hampton DC is a Doctor of Chiropractic who graduated from the Welsh Institute of Chiropractic in 2004 with a BSc (Hons) degree in Chiropractic. Louise has sat on the council of the British Chiropractic Association (BCA) and is a fellow of the BCA.

Over the past 14 years, Louise has treated hundreds of patients, easing their pain and making them feel better. Louise has found the people that have benefited most from treatment have tended to be those who also tried to help themselves through exercises and little changes to their lifestyle as well.

Usually, back pain comes on gradually, and it can be little things people do over time that add up to the pain. And it can be small things, like the exercises and pointers in this book that help alleviate the pain.

REVIEWS

"Chiropractor Louise Hampton has written a perfect book for chiropractors to have in their clinics for those that struggle with back pain. It is very informative yet easy to read and the recommended postural and exercises are brilliant. I can't wait to purchase this for Luck's Yard Clinic."

Tone Tellefsen Hughes DC, BSc, FRCC (paeds)

Chiropractor and Clinic owner

Luck's Yard Clinic

CONTENTS

ACKNOWLEDGEMENTS I
ABOUT THE AUTHOR II
REVIEWS III
INTRODUCTION 1
CHAPTER 1: ANATOMY OF THE LUMBAR SPINE 5
CHAPTER 2: NON-SPECIFIC LOW BACK PAIN 7
 RADICULAR PAIN AND RADICULOPATHY 8
 WEAR AND TEAR AND STENOSIS IN THE LOWER BACK 13
 HOW PAIN CAN AFFECT YOU 15
 YOUR MENTAL WELLBEING 16

CHAPTER 3: HOW TO HELP YOURSELF 19
 QUESTIONS TO ASK YOURSELF 19
 CHANGES TO TRY MAKING IN YOUR EVERYDAY LIFE 21

CHAPTER 4: HOW POSTURE AND LOAD AFFECTS THE SPINE 23
 THE EFFECT OF LIFTING A HEAVY LOAD ON THE DISC 25
 WHY IS BENDING BAD FOR THE BACK? 26
 CONSIDER WHAT IS HAPPENING TO THE DISCS AND HOW YOU CAN PREVENT AN INJURY 29
 HOW TO BEND CORRECTLY 31
 WAYS TO MOVE PAIN FREE IN BED 32
 HOW TO GET OUT OF BED IN THE MORNING 34

CHAPTER 5: ADVICE ON EVERYDAY ACTIVITIES 35

BEST WAY TO GET OUT OF A CHAIR 35

BEST WAYS TO LIFT 36

HOW TO STAND CORRECTLY 37

THINGS TO DO IF YOU HAVE TO STAND IN A QUEUE FOR A LONG TIME .. 39

HOW TO SIT CORRECTLY 43

HOW TO WALK TO HELP YOUR BACK 44

CHAPTER 6: CORE STABILITY 47

WHAT IS CORE STABILITY? 47

HOW TO ACTIVATE THE CORE MUSCLES 48

CHAPTER 7: THINGS TO DO TO HELP IF YOU HAVE SCIATICA OR A DISC PROLAPSE 51

HOW TO KEEP A DIARY 52

HOW TO KNOW IF YOUR PAIN IS GOING IN THE RIGHT DIRECTION 53

CHAPTER 8: EXERCISES TO TRY WHEN YOUR BACK IS BAD 55

STRETCHING THE GLUTEUS MUSCLES 60

MASSAGING THE GLUTEUS MUSCLES 61

NERVE FLOSSING 63

CHAPTER 9: CORE MUSCLE EXERCISES – (PILATES) 65

FIRST CORE MUSCLE EXERCISE 65

SECOND CORE MUSCLE EXERCISE 66

THIRD CORE MUSCLE EXERCISE 68

A GREAT WAY TO RELAX 69

CHAPTER 10: STRENGTHENING EXERCISES 71

CHAPTER 11: BALANCING EXERCISES 75

    ADVANCED BALANCING EXERCISES 79

CHAPTER 12: EXERCISES USING A FOAM ROLLER 81

CHAPTER 13: EXERCISES USING A SQUIDGY BALL 85

CHAPTER 14: PRODUCTS WHICH MIGHT HELP YOUR BACK PAIN 87

CHAPTER 15: TEN TOP TIPS TO HELP YOUR BACK 91

    TIP 1: BE CAREFUL WHEN YOU FIRST WAKE UP 91

    TIP 2: AVOID SLEEPING ON YOUR FRONT 92

    TIP 3: SLEEP WITH A PILLOW UNDER/BETWEEN YOUR LEGS 93

    TIP 4: AVOID LOTS OF BENDING 94

    TIP 5: HOLD YOUR PHONE UP 95

    TIP 6: WATCH YOUR POSTURE WHEN STANDING 96

    TIP 7: WALK TALL 97

    TIP 8: WEAR WELL-FITTING SHOES 98

    TIP 9: GO FOR A WALK 99

    TIP 10: KEEP HYDRATED 100

AND FINALLY… 101

REFERENCES 102

INTRODUCTION

This book has been written so that it is easy to understand but also incorporates a lot of different exercises based on expert advice. Everyone is different, and everyone's back pain is different, so there is no one exercise that will work for everyone. There are lots of different exercises in this book, and so hopefully you will be able to find some that suit you and your back. Research has shown there isn't one type of exercise which is best for back pain, the main thing is to find something you enjoy doing. If you have quite a sedentary lifestyle it is important to try and move more during the day.

If one exercise doesn't help, stop it and try another. It is also important to seek advice from a professional when it comes to back pain. There are a number of causes of back pain, and you need to make sure your pain is not being caused by something serious before you start an exercise routine. A chiropractor, osteopath or doctor can rule out serious causes of back pain - which fortunately, are very rare - and come to a diagnosis. Symptoms to look out for and get advice for include night pain, sweats and unexplained weight loss. Once you know your pain is definitely mechanical (i.e. coming from the muscles or joints) then combining exercises with some treatment will give your back the best chance of recovery.

Back pain may take time to get better, so don't despair. By thinking about how you sit and stand, and the impact different daily activities have on your spine, you can start to reduce the pressure on the low back, giving it a chance to heal. And to truly help the healing process, you can also look at what you eat and how stressed you are, as these factors contribute to the pain.

Got back pain? Feel like it's never going to go away? Or not sure what to do for the best? Please, don't panic. This book is designed to explain what could be causing your pain and to help you feel better.

I love to treat people, and I find it fascinating when I see patients in their nineties doing so well. What they all seem to have in common is that they are busy people who still exercise every day.

Back pain is very common. Most of us will suffer from it at some point in our lives, and as we are living longer, the number of people experiencing back pain is likely to increase (Hoy and colleagues, 2012). However, low back pain tends to subside within two to six weeks and by twelve weeks pain levels are low in most cases. Imaging such as an X-ray or MRI scan is rarely necessary. It is important to stay positive and try to keep moving.

As we get older, it is common to decrease the amount of exercise we do and start to slow down. Aches and pains, as well as injuries, occur more frequently too, making us want to exercise less often. However, the saying 'use it or lose it' is so true. It is more important than ever to keep moving, as the stronger and fitter we are, the better equipped the body is to deal with everyday life. Strength training is very important as we age, as our muscle strength tends to decrease with age.

In this book, I am going to go through the common causes of mechanical back pain to enable you to understand where the pain is coming from and how the body experiences pain. I will then give examples of stretches and routines you can do at home to stay fit and give examples of how people have overcome injuries to keep moving and stay as fit as possible, allowing them to get the most out of life.

This book explores all the different aspects of your life you can analyse to find out why your back pain started, and how you can get rid of the pain and stop it coming back, or at least manage the pain.

Over the years, I have come to notice how different everyone's pain is and how differently everyone responds to treatment. You could have three people with an MRI showing a disc bulge at L5/S1, but the level of pain they are experiencing or which orthopaedic tests show up as positive can vary considerably.

I have treated an athlete who could still touch her toes and had very minor neurological involvement despite the fact she had a significant prolapsed disc, and yet another patient with the same condition found it almost impossible to sit down, let alone touch her toes.

> When you have back pain, you find that everyone has an opinion on the best way to help it. They may have a good idea, but just remember that everyone responds differently – so just because something worked for them, it doesn't mean it will work for you.

The best thing you can do is listen to your body and find out what it likes and doesn't like to do. Most backs do not like bending or lifting heavy objects, but with exercises it is very much a matter of trial and error to find out which positions suit you best and help to prevent your pain returning. Keep trying to stay positive and remember that the pain is very likely to go – it will just take a bit of time.

CHAPTER 1: ANATOMY OF THE LUMBAR SPINE

This section provides some details of the anatomy of the low back, which should help to give you a better understanding of your back.

The low back is made up of five vertebrae named L1 - L5. These are designed to support loads and bear the weight of the rest of the spine. The intervertebral discs are in between each vertebra and these help to absorb shocks and distribute weight. When you bend forward the pressure in the discs increases considerably. As we get older the size of the discs reduces, and therefore you can feel extra pressure on the bones and joints in the spine causing them to be stiff and achy.

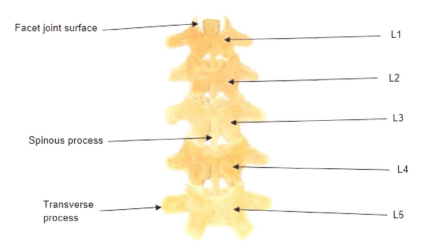

Figure 1: Lumbar vertebrae, posterior view.

Muscles and ligaments surround the spine to hold the spine together and enable it to move. In a healthy back there is a balance between muscles acting to protect the spine from excessive movement and still allowing normal movement to occur. Most of the time it is not possible to identify exactly what is causing the pain in the back. There are only a small number of known causes such as a fracture, cancer or infection but these are very rare. The majority of causes are grouped together as non-specific low back pain (Hartvigsen and colleagues, 2018).

With low back pain it is common to feel tenderness in the spine and for the muscles in the area to become tight. Sometimes trigger points which are small areas of muscle which have gone into spasm can be felt. These can cause decreased blood flow to the area, with pain and restricted movement.

CHAPTER 2: NON-SPECIFIC LOW BACK PAIN

Low back pain is a symptom and is usually taken to be where you are getting the pain, from the lower rib margins to the buttock creases and can also include pain into one or both legs or include neurological symptoms in the lower limbs. It is rarely possible to find the main cause of the low back pain. Low back pain tends to have many dimensions from the biophysical component to the psychological and then the social impact as well.

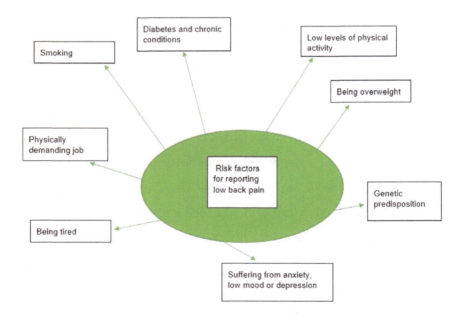

Figure 2: Low back pain contributing factors. Information taken from Hartvigsen and colleagues, 2018.

RADICULAR PAIN AND RADICULOPATHY

Radicular pain is when pain is felt in one of the legs due to compression of a nerve root. The leg pain tends to be worse than the back pain and it can be diagnosed by performing a straight leg-raise test and Valsalva manoeuvre (which is where it is painful to cough, sneeze and strain). Radiculopathy is when the nerve root compression causes weakness in a leg muscle, the loss of a reflex or loss of sensation relating to a particular nerve root. Radicular pain and radiculopathy can occur together, and one of the most common causes is a disc herniation with inflammation.

The discs are in the spine between each of the vertebra. They cushion the spine and are made up of a fibrous outer layer with a centre made of a jelly type substance. With a lumbar disc prolapse, some of the outer fibres of the disc tear, causing the disc to press against a nerve. When the nerve is aggravated, it causes pain down one or both of the legs. This is usually a problem for people under 60. It can also be called a slipped disc or a cause of sciatica. Usually, the discs are not seen by the body, so when a disc protrudes the body starts to attack it as if it were foreign, increasing the inflammation in the area and therefore the pressure on the nerve root.

A good way to think of the disc is like a jam doughnut where the nucleus pulposus is the jam in the middle that gets pushed out.

Remember: if the pain goes down both legs, you have numbness in the saddle region (around the anus) and you experience urinary retention (not being able to pass urine) sometimes with overflow incontinence, then you must seek immediate medical help. This, however, is extremely rare.

When the disc is involved, the pain can be quite severe. Quite often it is worse in the morning, when the discs contain the most water. (As the day goes on water is pressed out of the discs, so you are generally 1–2 centimetres shorter at the end of the day.) You can also experience numbness in a leg or foot and tingling as the nerve is compressed.

Lumbar disc prolapse can cause extreme pain in the back and leg. The good news is that 80% of patients with prolapsed discs recover within around six weeks, so it is important to remain positive.

Going to work and still going out socially are really important, as doing so helps you both physically and mentally. Back pain can get you down, but if you are aware of this then you can look out for it and do things to help both your physical and mental health.

Further on in this book, I will detail some specific exercises you can try to help reduce the pressure on the sciatic nerve.

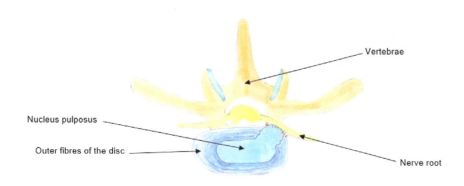

Figure 3: A slice through the spine showing the nerves and disc. See how the outer fibres have torn allowing the nucleus to come out and press against the nerve along with inflammation.

Staying positive, still going to work and doing exercise are extremely important when you have low back pain.

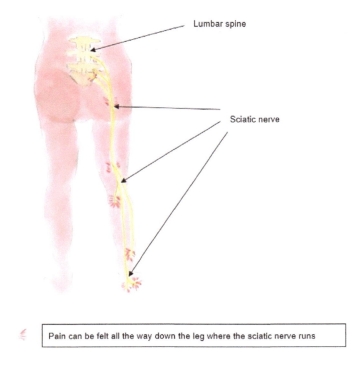

Pain can be felt all the way down the leg where the sciatic nerve runs

Figure 4: The sciatic nerve from where it leaves the spine. See how when the nerve is compressed in the spine with inflammation it can cause pain all the way down the path of the nerve into the foot. The more the nerve is compressed the further down the leg you will feel the pain. In some instances, instead of pain you can have tingling or numbness into the leg and foot.

Treatment from a chiropractor can include the use of blocks (two wedges that you lie on) to realign the pelvis and reduce the tension on the discs, flexion/distraction as a way of mobilising the joints, massage to help the muscle tension, manipulation and home exercises to strengthen the back. A study by Lewis and colleagues (2015) showed manipulation as well as acupuncture to be effective forms of treatment for sciatica and should be considered as part of a treatment package.

WEAR AND TEAR AND STENOSIS IN THE LOWER BACK

As we get older, the discs narrow, and we can get a little bit of bony growth from the vertebra (osteophytes). Most people just feel a bit of stiffness in the spine, but some feel pain going into the leg and struggle to walk long distances.

Do you find it easier to walk with a shopping trolley? Or can you only walk a short distance before feeling pain in your back? These are just some of the questions a therapist would ask to help diagnose stenosis in the spine.

Although a chiropractor is unable to cure wear and tear in the spine, improving the function of the spine means that movement can be increased, and pain can be reduced. So, it is definitely worth giving a chiropractor a try.

One recent study by Ammendolia and colleagues, (2018) has shown following an intensive six week programme of chiropractic care, patients were able to walk a further 500 metres.

How to help eliminate low back pain and achieve long term relief

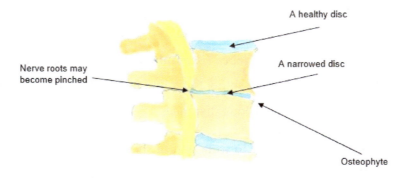

Figure 5: Lateral view of the spine showing stenosis.

HOW PAIN CAN AFFECT YOU

Pain is a symptom we are still trying to understand. At a cellular level nerve cells called neurons transmit impulses down a nerve. The inside of the cell is usually negatively charged however, when an impulse is sent from a cell body, sodium ions flood into the cell and the impulse is transmitted down the nerve through a series of action potentials. Usually neurons do not fire an action potential unless stimulated to do so. When a nerve is injured however, it can repeatedly fire and become hypersensitive. Or it can sit just under the threshold, so that the slightest thing makes the neuron fire, such as a small movement, extra stress or heat.

Many things play a part in the pain process. You may have pain in your leg one hour but not the next. Or sometimes you can be tickled and sometimes not. There are so many things that can affect the outcome.

Pain can be seen as a circular model, where the pain can start anywhere along the circle and can be changed by the different inputs and feedback. The following figure shows how so many things impact pain.

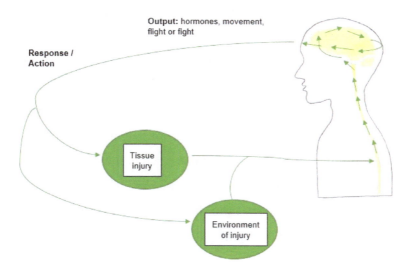

Figure 6: Circular model of pain. Adapted from the book by Butler (2000). (Original from Gifford LS (1998) Pain, the tissues and the nervous system. Physiotherapy 84:27 - 33).

YOUR MENTAL WELLBEING

Being in pain can get you down, so it is more important than ever to try to remain positive and keep your stress levels down.

Looking at your mental wellbeing is extremely important. Studies have shown that cognitive behavioural therapy (CBT) and mindfulness-based stress reduction (MBSR) are excellent ways to help you deal with the pain (Turner and colleagues 2016).

CBT is a talking therapy which helps change how you think and behave so that you can cope with the pain. MBSR was developed at a university in America and usually combines mindfulness meditation with yoga and body awareness. It tends to be an eight week programme, and it can also help you cope with and manage pain better (Cherkin and colleagues 2016).

If you don't want to see someone or go to a group meeting there is also a lot of help online these days. The website www.bemindfulonline.com offers an online course that enables you to practise mindfulness and I am sure there is a lot of other information on You Tube.

An app on the website www.curablehealth.com is a great way to help chronic pain. If you have been in pain for more than a few months this app is definitely worth a try.

Practising meditation and mindfulness is such a great way to help relax the body. When the body experiences pain, it can become hypersensitive and the slightest thing can make the pain worse. By practising things like mindfulness, you help tone down the hypersensitivity.

There is a great book called *The Miracle Morning* which walks you through things to do before eight a.m. to get your day off to a good start. It includes saying affirmations, doing some meditation, and exercise, and writing in a journal. This could be a great place to start, and then you can develop the mindfulness and meditation further. Being positive makes such a difference.

How to help eliminate low back pain and achieve long term relief

CHAPTER 3: HOW TO HELP YOURSELF

QUESTIONS TO ASK YOURSELF

If you experience back pain it is important to look at what you do in your everyday life that might be aggravating your back.

- Do you spend a lot of time sitting?
- Do you have to carry heavy loads?
- Do you have to bend a lot?
- Do you spend a lot of time driving?
- Are you overweight?
- Do you sleep on your front?
- Do you look after small children?
- Have you had an accident or jarred your back in the past?
- Do you play any impact sports?
- No time for myself?
- Am I stressed?

If you answered 'yes' to any of these questions, that might be what is contributing to your back pain.

On the next page are some ideas of changes you could try making in your everyday life, to see if they can ease your pain or stop it returning.

CHANGES TO TRY MAKING IN YOUR EVERYDAY LIFE

- Could you get up and walk about every hour? Set a timer so that you are reminded to get up and move. If you are engrossed in something, it is very easy to not notice time passing, and before you know it, two hours could have passed without you moving.

- Could you lie down for five minutes now and again? That would really take the pressure off the spine during the day.

- Could you decrease the load you carry or wear a support belt? Try to avoid lifting with a bad back, as this will aggravate it further. If your job involves lifting, look at purchasing a support belt to wear just when you have to lift something heavy.

- Could you bend from your hips? Bending puts a lot of pressure on the spine, so if you can change how you bend – and avoid doing so where possible – this could make a real difference. See the section on bending for more information.

- Could you take breaks from driving to walk about? Try not to drive for more than two hours without taking a break to move around. When you are driving, try clenching your buttocks and wriggling in your seat to get the blood flowing to your muscles.

- Could you look at what you eat and reduce your calorie intake? Carrying extra weight can put extra pressure on your spine. Be honest with yourself, and if you are overweight look at reducing what you eat. Try joining a group like Weight Watchers for support.

- Could you change your sleeping position? Consider how you sleep. Sleeping on your side or back is preferable to sleeping on your front.

- Could you try some strengthening exercises for your back, to help it recover from an injury? You can do strengthening exercises in the long term once the initial pain has subsided.

- Could you reduce your training to give your back a chance to recover? If you're an athlete or in training, when your back is bad, ease off the training to give your back a chance to recover.

- Look at making time for yourself and ways to destress. Your mental health is very important. Look into meditation and mindfulness you will be surprised the difference it can make.

CHAPTER 4: HOW POSTURE AND LOAD AFFECTS THE SPINE

We all know that sitting for a long time can be bad for the back. But do you know how much pressure the spine is put under depending on the position you are in? Look at how sitting puts more pressure on the spine than standing.

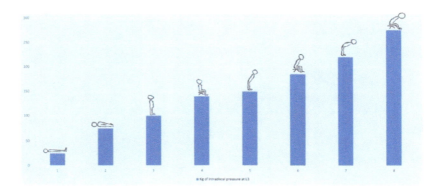

Figure 7: Pressure exerted on the lumbar discs in different postures (based on Nachemson, 1966). This diagram shows loading (in kilograms) recorded by intradiscal pressure transducers inserted into the L3 disc space of volunteers. Not many realise that there is more loading in the sitting, rather than the standing, position. Even when lying down, there remains some loading on the spine.

Floating in water can be an excellent way of taking the pressure off the spine, as you do not have gravity causing pressure on the spine. Special devices have been made over the years to help keep you floating in the water, and these could be great if you have back pain and just want to reduce the load on the discs for a while.

Just try to make some small changes, like how you get up from a chair or losing a bit of weight, and you will be surprised at the difference it can make. How about just lying on your back during an advert break? Give it a try.

THE EFFECT OF LIFTING A HEAVY LOAD ON THE DISC.

Any lifting you do puts pressure on the discs. If, however you already have back pain coming from a suspected prolapse and you lift a weight you are likely to make the problem worse. As you can see in the diagram the disc is put under a lot more pressure when a weight is applied, and this can lead to further inflammation and pain.

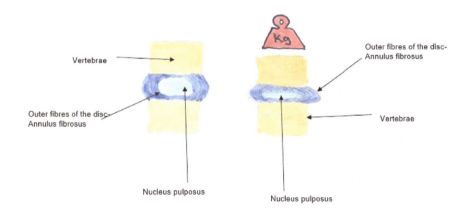

Figure 8: What happens to the lumbar disc with load. Adapted from an illustration by Jasper Baeke.

In this diagram, you can see how the fibres of the annulus fibrosus are stretched as the weight is applied. This is how little micro-tears can occur. Prolonged pressure on the discs increases the chances of the fibres tearing. It is therefore important when doing exercises to protect the spine that we focus on endurance not just strength, so we do more repetitions of a lower weight rather than lifting anything heavy.

In the morning, the discs typically have a greater water content and are more prone to injury. Avoid any spinal exercises when you first get up, especially those where you bend the spine, as this puts extra pressure on the discs. This is why it can be a lot more difficult to put socks on in the morning than it is to take them off in the evening. Over the course of the day, the pressure of gravity pushing down on the discs causes water to leave the discs and so the discs narrow. This can mean you are around 2 centimetres taller in the morning than at night.

Lying down for longer than eight hours can also stress the spine. It causes extra pressure on the discs caused by the increased water content, McGill (2002).

WHY IS BENDING BAD FOR THE BACK?

Think about a paperclip: you can bend it forward and back, forward and back, and eventually it goes snap. The back is not that dissimilar. The discs in the back get aggravated by bending, so after a while tiny tears start to occur in the outer fibres of the disc, and eventually it herniates, just like the paperclip that breaks.

As can be seen from Figure 7 just bending forward a little bit when standing puts 50 kilograms of extra force through the spine, so it doubles the pressure on the spine – which over time can lead to injury.

If you repeatedly aggravate an area, a problem can build up. Say your new shoes rub on your feet. Over time, just the slightest touch of the shoe can cause pain. It is the same for the back. If you repeatedly bend it, soon it won't take much to cause pain, as the area becomes hypersensitive.

Injury to the spine doesn't have to be one major event. Most commonly, it is a build-up of minor things, like sitting at a desk all day or bending a lot when you do the housework. If you are in one position long enough, tiny tears will occur, which will lead to an injury.

How you bend the spine has a massive impact on the pressure put through it. If you bend your spine to pick something up, there can be over 100 times more pressure put through the spine than if you keep your back straight. Picture 'a' is putting far more pressure through the spine than picture 'b'. Adapted from McGill (2002).

(See following diagrams).

How to help eliminate low back pain and achieve long term relief

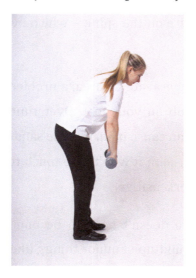

a.

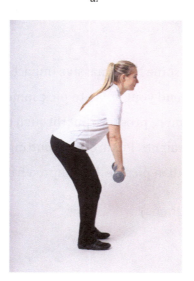

b.

CONSIDER WHAT IS HAPPENING TO THE DISCS AND HOW YOU CAN PREVENT AN INJURY

As already discussed, the discs have more water content first thing in the morning, so this is a time when you must be extra careful about bending and lifting.

The same applies when you have been in one position for a long time. For example, if you have spent a long time sitting in a car, the ligaments around the spine will have stretched and loosened, and there will have been a lot of stress on the discs, possibly causing some micro-tears. If you then go to lift something heavy without giving the ligaments a chance to stiffen and the discs a chance to recover, then an injury is more likely to occur.

If you know you must drive to a job where lifting is involved, you can wear either a back support in the car or have a lumbar roll on your seat to try to keep your back in extension, so there is less pressure on the discs.

By thinking about what pressure your back is put through and trying to change position when you can, the risk of injuries can be minimised.

A back support could also be worn if you have experienced back pain in the past but must lift as part of your job. Back supports are not recommended if you have never had back pain, but they can help if you have had pain in the past. They should only be worn for short periods, though.

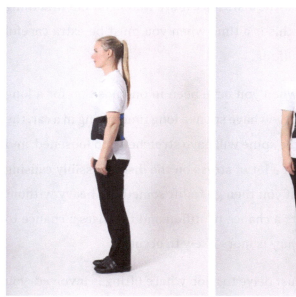

If you work in an office, it is hard to pay attention to how often you get up, especially if you are busy. Make sure you drink a lot of water, as then you will need to get up frequently to go to the toilet. Set an alarm on your watch or phone for fifty minutes, so that you can spend five minutes an hour actively stretching and moving. Also, use your lunch break to go for a walk. This will be so helpful both mentally and physically.

HOW TO BEND CORRECTLY

The best way to bend is from the hips, not the spine. Our hips are designed to bend a lot and easily, so it is important that we use them.

First, stand up tall and place your hands on your thighs. Next, slowly move your hands down your thighs to your knees, whilst sticking your bottom out. This will mean your back will remain straight as you go to sit down rather than your back bending. This will protect your back.

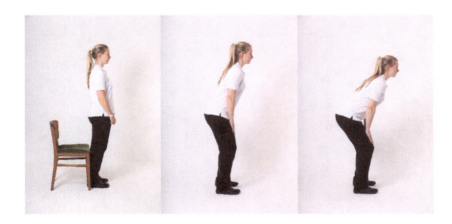

WAYS TO MOVE PAIN FREE IN BED

If you are finding it very painful to turn in bed, see if this can help.

To roll over when you are on one side, stiffen your core muscles by gently pulling your tummy in. Lift up the top arm and leg quickly, which will then help you to roll over – by keeping your core strong as you do so, your back will be protected. Adapted from McGill (2002).

(See following diagrams).

CHAPTER 4: HOW POSTURE AND LOAD AFFECTS THE SPINE

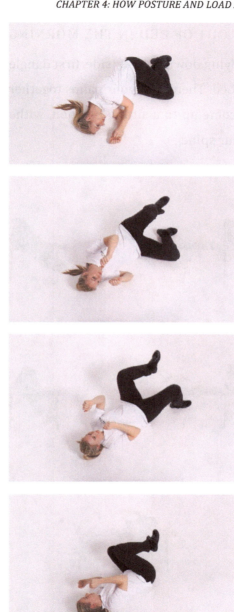

33

HOW TO GET OUT OF BED IN THE MORNING

To sit up from lying down on your side, first dangle your legs over the end of the bed. Then push your palms together. This will help you naturally come up to a sitting position, without putting any pressure on your spine.

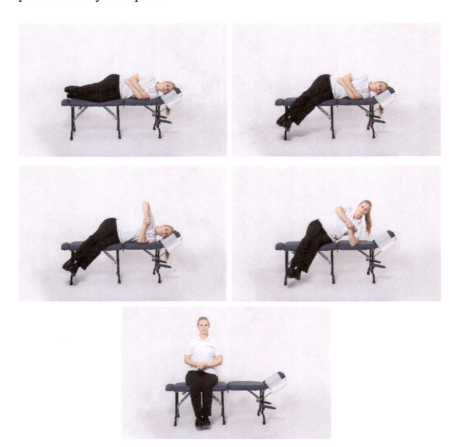

CHAPTER 5: ADVICE ON EVERYDAY ACTIVITIES

BEST WAY TO GET OUT OF A CHAIR

Rather than bending your back when getting out of a chair, try to stick your bottom out and keep your spine straight. This avoids bending the spine and prevents further pressure on the spine. Think back to the paperclip: every time you get out of a chair and bend your spine, it's like bending the paperclip forward and back, making the chances of your back giving way greater. As getting out of a chair is something you do many times a day, by just changing this habit, you can really help strengthen your spine. You can use the same technique when lowering into a chair as well.

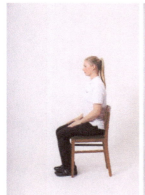
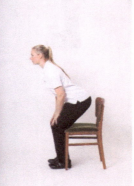
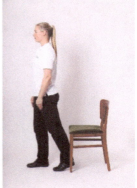

BEST WAYS TO LIFT

Remember to keep a straight back and bend from the hips when picking up anything heavy. If you are reaching to pick up something light, you can lift one leg in the air and keep the back straight as you go down.

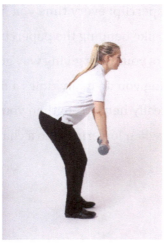

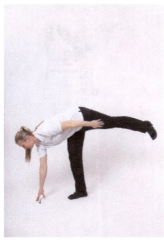

HOW TO STAND CORRECTLY

If you must stand for any length of time, it is common for your back to start hurting. When standing, try to contract your core muscles to provide a corset of support around your spine. Think also of being pulled up by the top of your head.

Look at the difference here between good and bad posture – so much more pressure is being put through the entire spine when in bad posture. When looking at posture the main thing to also consider is to change position frequently as if you stay in any posture long enough it will be bad for the back. The main thing is to keep moving.

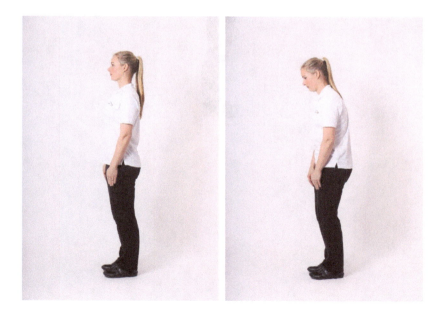

An example of good posture   *An example of bad posture*

This is a stretch to try. We tend to spend a long time with our arms forward in life either at a computer or looking at a phone. Try to have your thumbs pointing outwards, as this will keep your shoulders back. Tuck your chin in, and relax your knees (locking knees puts pressure on them).

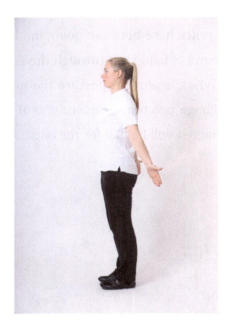

CHAPTER 5: ADVICE ON EVERYDAY ACTIVITIES

THINGS TO DO IF YOU HAVE TO STAND IN A QUEUE FOR A LONG TIME

Try putting your hands in the small of your back and leaning backwards slightly to take the pressure off the discs. Just hold this position for a few seconds and then repeat every few minutes, so long as it is not painful to do. Sometimes leaning backwards can be painful especially if the joints in your back are inflamed. If this is the case, then try bending forwards instead to flex the spine and take the pressure off the joints.

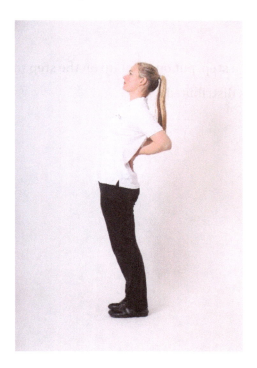

How to help eliminate low back pain and achieve long term relief

Try moving your hips from side to side. If the pressure is constantly in the same place that is when the back will hurt more.

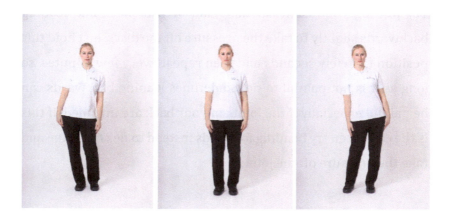

If you are near a step, put one foot up on the step to change where the pressure is distributed.

CHAPTER 5: ADVICE ON EVERYDAY ACTIVITIES

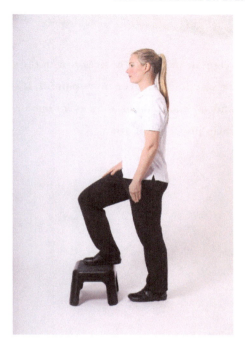

Standing can be uncomfortable for most people, but if you have back pain you are bound to notice your back more if you must stand in a queue for any length of time. The important thing to do is to try to keep moving – even if that means just shifting from one leg to the other, forwards and backwards. This will help keep the blood flowing. Clenching your buttocks in the queue is also worth a try.

How to help eliminate low back pain and achieve long term relief

If you are overweight or pregnant the pressure on the spine is increased, and this can make standing still even more painful. If you know you will be standing around say shopping or at an event maybe look at wearing a back support to help just for that event.

HOW TO SIT CORRECTLY

Sitting for long periods of time should be avoided if possible. But if you have to sit – for a long journey, for example – here are a few things to try:

Clench your buttocks or move in your seat, to get the blood circulating to the muscles.

Put a lumbar support cushion behind your back.

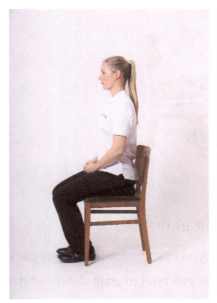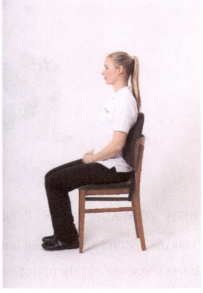

If that doesn't suit your back, see if a wedge cushion is more comfortable.

Try moving to the edge of the seat and have one leg forward and one back. This can make sitting upright more effortless, and as you are less likely to slouch, there will be less pressure on the discs.

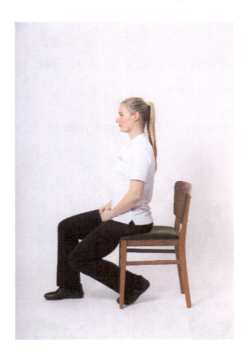

HOW TO WALK TO HELP YOUR BACK

This may sound strange, but have you ever noticed that your back hurts if you are out shopping, when you tend to walk slowly whilst browsing, and yet a brisk walk can normally help your back? This is because when you walk more quickly, you tend to use your arms, which means muscles in your back are being used, which in turn reduces the pressure on the spine.

CHAPTER 5: ADVICE ON EVERYDAY ACTIVITIES

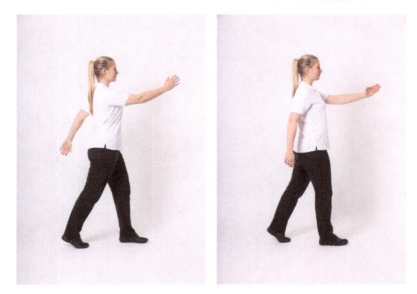

Because of this, next time you are out shopping, try swinging your arms from your shoulders, and you should find that your back is more comfortable. McGill (2002).

How to help eliminate low back pain and achieve long term relief

CHAPTER 6: CORE STABILITY

With low back pain it is very common for the muscles around the spine to weaken especially your core muscles. Exercise like Pilates can be a fantastic way to strengthen your back in a gentle way.

WHAT IS CORE STABILITY?

Core stability is how the muscles around the spine support and protect it. Core muscles act a bit like a corset around the spine providing support from all sides. It is important that this system is engaged before movement begins so that the low back can remain stable whilst the rest of the body moves. After you have been contracting the core muscles for a period of time, using your core muscles becomes a natural reaction.

It can take some time to learn how to activate and contract the core muscles. There are a couple of ways to think about activating the core muscles – see which one works for you. You can either think of tightening your stomach when trying to fit into a pair of jeans or going away from an ice cube on your tummy. The contraction should be slow and mild at around 50% of your effort.

HOW TO ACTIVATE THE CORE MUSCLES

Contracting the core muscles does take some getting used to and it can seem quite complicated at first, but don't give up!

Start off by lying on your back with the knees bent. Put your fingers on your pelvic bone (the bone that protrudes just by the hips) and slide them along the bone 1–2 centimetres towards the middle of the abdomen. The muscle you are trying to activate runs left to right from one hip to the other.

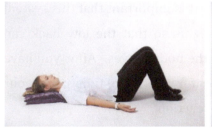 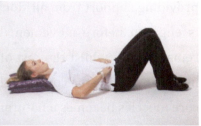

Pull your tummy in and downwards towards your coccyx (sitting bone), pulling this muscle flat. You should feel a bulge under your fingers as the muscle activates. The back should not move and your stomach should not hollow. All you should feel is this muscle tightening.

Remember, it is a slow, mild contraction with 50% effort.

The same muscle is used when you cough, so you can cough to make sure you are contracting the right muscle. Pain when coughing and sneezing is also a common symptom in people whose core muscles have become weak.

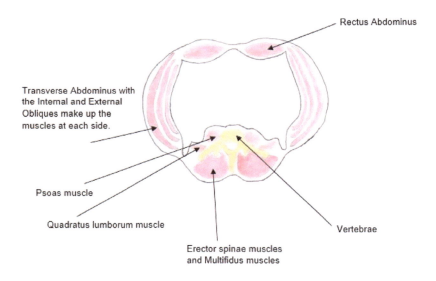

Figure 9: Diagram showing the muscles providing the corset of support around the spine (adapted from McGill, 2002).

How to help eliminate low back pain and achieve long term relief

CHAPTER 7: THINGS TO DO TO HELP IF YOU HAVE SCIATICA OR A DISC PROLAPSE

- Try using an ice pack. The area can become very inflamed with a prolapsed disc and using an ice pack can help calm the inflammation down. Wrap an ice pack in a tea towel and lie on it for around five minutes at a time to numb the area. Repeat every hour when your back is at its worst.

- Change position every 15 to 20 minutes. It is easy for your back to become stiff and lock up when it is inflamed. By changing position, you help to keep it more mobile. Lying down will mean less pressure through the discs. When it is very bad move from lying on your back with your knees bent to lying on your side with a pillow between your knees and then try a small amount of time on your front. Once the pain starts to decrease slightly then try to spend five minutes at a time gently walking.

- Avoid lifting and bending. Both put tremendous pressure on the discs and if they are inflamed then just carrying something light can be enough to set the pain off again. No hoovering, washing up or mowing the lawn either as the slight bending when you are doing these tasks is enough to aggravate the back.

- Look at your diet and avoid foods that cause more inflammation such as sugar and grains. Look up a diet that reduces inflammation. Turmeric is also a great supplement to take to reduce inflammation.

- Twisting to get out of a car can be painful so put a plastic bag on the seat and that will make it easier to turn.

- If you are sitting to watch T.V. make sure your back is supported and that your hips are higher than your knees. Wedge cushions can be quite useful. If you are sitting in a deep sofa and your feet do not reach the floor, make sure you have a foot rest. Try using a lumbar roll behind your back too. It's all about finding a position that is comfortable.

- If you need to cough or sneeze avoid bending forward at the same time. Instead stand up and bend backwards slightly as this will reduce the pressure on the discs.

- Take a look at your mental health. Are you particularly stressed or depressed? This can affect your back pain and your recovery.

HOW TO KEEP A DIARY

When keeping a diary, try to note down how you felt in yourself that day – whether you were particularly tired or had lots of energy. Write down times when you experienced pain and what you were doing. For example, note if you felt some pain when getting out of a chair or when you stood in a queue. Also note down any good times or times when you had no pain. Try to rate your pain out of 10, with 1 being next to no pain and 10 being the worst pain imaginable.

By keeping a diary, you might be able to see whether certain activities aggravate your back. The diary can also show you how you are improving, even though it might not feel like you are making much progress. Over time, you are looking for the number of good times to increase. Back pain tends to be very much up and down, so don't worry if the pain returns for the odd day. The main thing is that overall the amount of pain is decreasing.

It is also important to set some realistic goals for how and when you will do your exercises and to have a milestone to aim for, like being able to walk for ten minutes without pain after a month. Try setting goals with a health practitioner to keep you motivated, and they can make sure the goals are realistic and achievable.

Trying to keep positive is very important when you have back pain. It is very easy to become down or depressed when you are in a lot of pain. If you do think you are getting depressed, try to talk to your doctor and get some help as stress and depression can also impact on how quickly you recover.

Try also to still go out and meet up with friends. Maybe join a pilates class or meditation group, talking through your problems and being around friends is also important. Froud (2013.)

HOW TO KNOW IF YOUR PAIN IS GOING IN THE RIGHT DIRECTION

If you have been experiencing pain in the back and down the leg, then as the back starts to heal, the pain in the leg should reduce and it should become more centralised in the low back (see Figure

10). If this does not happen when you follow the exercises in this book, then it is important to seek advice.

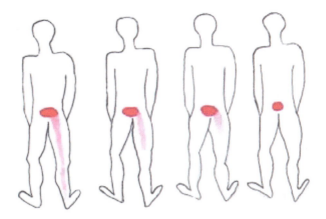

Figure 10: Caption (adapted from McKenzie, 2011).

CHAPTER 8: EXERCISES TO TRY WHEN YOUR BACK IS BAD

Here are some exercises to try to help with sciatica or a disc problem.

Lying on your front can sometimes provide relief if you have a problem with a disc, as it pushes the disc away from the nerve. It doesn't help everyone, but it is a position worth trying. (If it doesn't relieve your symptoms, though, then stop this exercise. No exercise should cause pain, and if any exercise does, you must stop and seek advice.)

The following exercises are adapted from the McKenzie Method, as outlined in the book *Treat Your Own Back* (McKenzie, 2011).

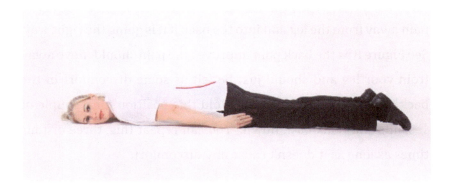

When you first lie on your front, just try to let your low back relax and sink down, creating a slight dip in your low back. This maybe uncomfortable for a few seconds as the joints go back into each other but then it should ease. If it doesn't feel a bit better, stop this exercise and do not progress to the next one- your back is not ready for this yet. Make sure you seek advice.

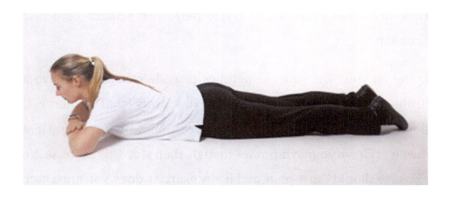

If you found it comfortable to lie on your front you can then try raising your head and coming up slightly. This will increase the dip in the low back and take even more pressure off the discs. Again, this should not be painful to do and should help to draw the pain away from the leg and into the back if it is going the right way. See Figure 8 as the back pain improves the pain should move away from your leg and should just be felt as some discomfort in the back before going completely. Hold this position for a couple of seconds and relax back down. You can repeat this, three or four times as long as it doesn't cause any discomfort.

CHAPTER 8: EXERCISES TO TRY WHEN YOUR BACK IS BAD

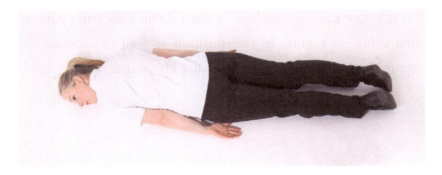

If lying on your front is okay but you are still experiencing a bit of discomfort into the leg then try shifting your pelvis away from the leg pain.

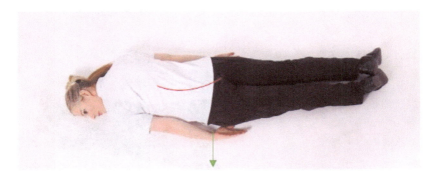

If the pain you experience is down the right leg, try shifting your hips over to the left. This can be another way to take the pressure away from where the disc is pressing. As you can see from the pictures it doesn't have to be a big movement but even moving this much can help some people so it is worth a try.

If it is easier having your hips to one side on your front you can then come up slightly in this position as well to increase the stretch further and take more pressure off the disc.

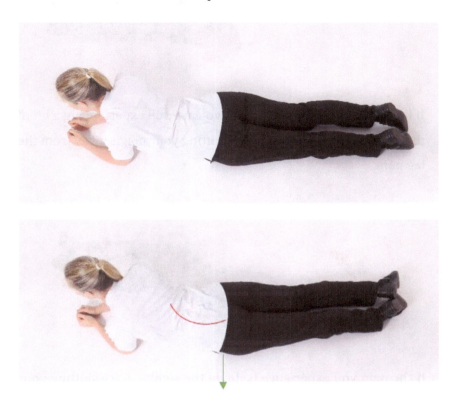

Once your back is very comfortable with the exercises you can come right up. Hold for just a couple of seconds.

CHAPTER 8: EXERCISES TO TRY WHEN YOUR BACK IS BAD

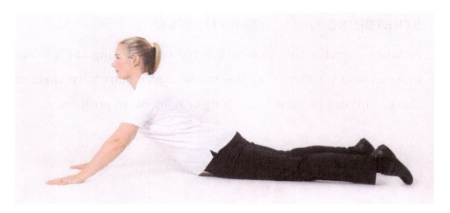

Do these exercises slowly and carefully, and remember, they should not be painful to do. Only hold a position for a couple of seconds and then relax back down again. You can repeat the exercises a few times in one session, and perform them a few times a day if you find them relieving.

How to help eliminate low back pain and achieve long term relief

STRETCHING THE GLUTEUS MUSCLES

Another exercise that is worth a try is stretching the gluteus muscles and piriformis as the sciatic nerve runs very close to these. This can be done in a sitting or lying down position.

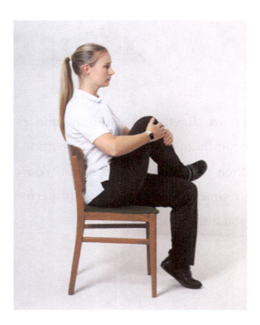

When sitting, cross one leg in front of you and pull the knee towards your chest to feel the stretch in the buttock. Hold this stretch for 10 to 15 seconds.

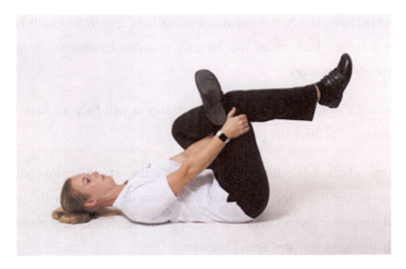

Lie down and bend both knees up. Rest one ankle on the other knee so it looks like a figure 4. Next gently pull the bottom leg towards you. You should feel the stretch in the buttock.

Try this exercise in both positions and see whether one is more comfortable to do. Repeat this exercise three times on both legs. The sciatic nerve runs very close to the buttock muscles and so if these muscles are tight it can put extra pressure on the nerve. This exercise should help to relieve some of the tension on the nerve.

MASSAGING THE GLUTEUS MUSCLES

With back pain it is very common for the muscles in the buttocks to be so tight that even with some stretching it is very hard to get them to relax.

How to help eliminate low back pain and achieve long term relief

Another way to try to stop them going into spasm so much is to use a spikey ball under the buttock muscles to essentially give yourself a massage.

If you do this for five minutes every day it will help to ease the spasm and reduce the pain.

To use a ball under the gluteus muscles either stand against a wall or lie on the floor and move gently backwards and forwards or up and down on the ball to gently massage the muscles. This exercise will also help the piriformis muscle.

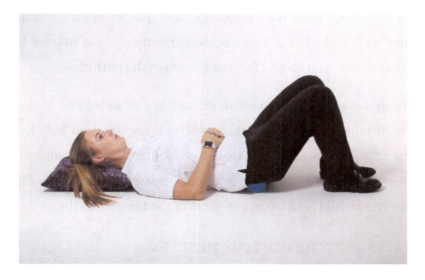

It is quite easy to purchase a spikey ball on online or any soft ball would be fine to use. If it is too hard like a golf ball it may be too painful to use.

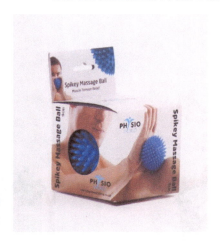

NERVE FLOSSING

If you have tight hamstrings the temptation is to stretch them, but this can aggravate the sciatic nerve. In his book *The Sensitive Nervous System* (2000), David Butler explains that the best way to help relieve the tension on the sciatic nerve is to do something called nerve flossing. Nerve flossing can help take the pressure off the sciatic nerve by mobilising the nerve from the surrounding soft tissues, relieving the pressure on the nerve.

You start bent over, with your knees bent, and then lean backwards as you straighten out one leg. This should not be painful to do and should help reduce the tension on the sciatic nerve. If it is painful to do, stop and seek advice.

How to help eliminate low back pain and achieve long term relief

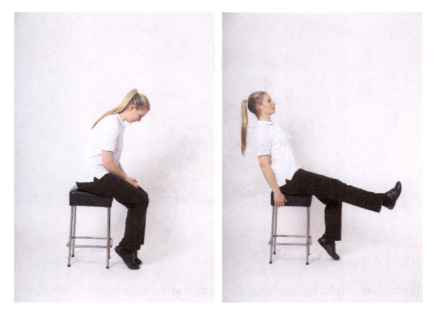

The most important thing with sciatica or a disc problem is to seek advice. Find out exactly what's wrong by seeing a physiotherapist, osteopath or chiropractor who can go through a full examination and then come up with a treatment plan. By combining exercises and treatment you will make a quicker recovery.

CHAPTER 9: CORE MUSCLE EXERCISES – (PILATES)

Here are three different exercises to try slowly to help strengthen your back. It is important to remain relaxed when performing these exercises, only contracting the core muscles. These exercises should not be painful to perform so if you do experience pain please seek professional advice.

FIRST CORE MUSCLE EXERCISE

Lie on the floor on your back with your knees bent and your core gently contracted. As you breathe out slowly bring one leg out to an imaginary two o'clock. Then as you breathe in take the leg back again, keeping all other muscles relaxed. Then try doing the same on the other side.

Remember to stay relaxed; only your core muscles should be contracting. Try to concentrate on breathing slowly and deeply.

It will take some time to learn to control your breathing and keep all your other muscles relaxed when doing this exercise.

How to help eliminate low back pain and achieve long term relief

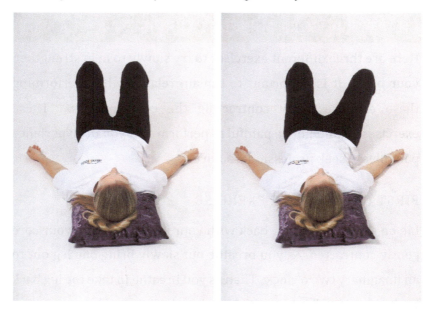

SECOND CORE MUSCLE EXERCISE

First just relax on your side. Try to think about all your muscles relaxing and switching off. The only contracting muscle should be in your tummy.

CHAPTER 9: CORE MUSCLE EXERCISES – (PILATES)

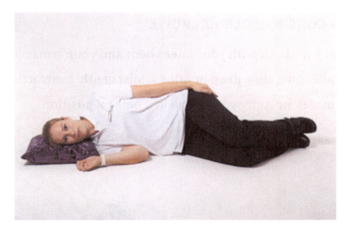

Lying on your side lift up your top leg keeping your feet together and your core gently contracting. Hold at the top for five seconds then gently lower. You should try to co-ordinate this exercise with your breathing so when you breathe out you raise the leg up and as you breathe in you lower the leg back down. Repeat on the other side.

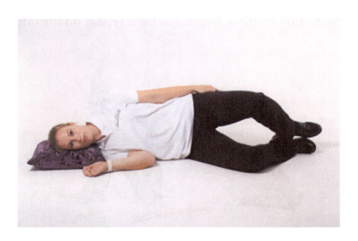

THIRD CORE MUSCLE EXERCISE

Relax on your back with your knees bent and your arms out to the side. Take some slow deep breaths whilst gently contracting your core muscles, keeping your spine in a neutral position.

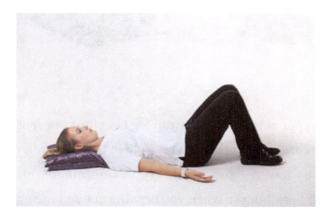

From this position as you breathe out slowly lift one leg up into a table top position. Then as you breathe in slowly lower the leg back down. Do this three times and then repeat on the other side.

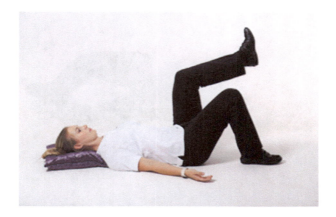

A GREAT WAY TO RELAX

Simply lying on the floor with a small cushion under your head can be a great position in which to relax and give your back and neck a rest. When you rest in this position, the pressure on the spine is greatly reduced. This is ideal for the evening when watching television. Just lie down for around five to minutes at a time and you will notice a big difference in how your back feels.

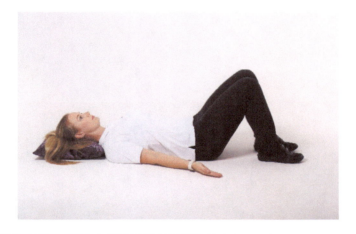

This is such a great way to help the back. Try this for just five or ten minutes every evening and it will make a big difference to your spine.

How to help eliminate low back pain and achieve long term relief

CHAPTER 10: STRENGTHENING EXERCISES

Once your back feels less vulnerable and you are able to do the core exercises with ease you can then move on to strengthening your back further. If you do strengthening exercises every evening, you help keep your back strong once it has recovered. Combining these exercises with a Pilates course would be a fantastic way to help your back in the long term.

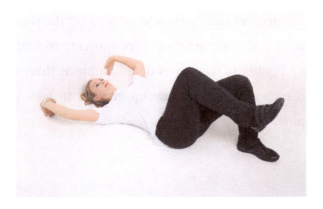

With your hands pressed against a wall, slowly raise one leg off the ground with a bent knee and then put it back down. Repeat with the other leg so it is like you are marching with your feet as you continue to press against the wall. You should feel a slight stretch down your back but no pain. Do this exercise for thirty seconds building up to three sets.

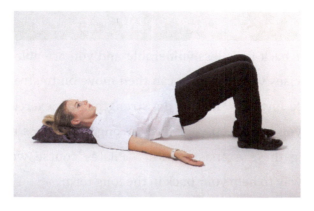

Lying on the ground slowly raise your hips off the floor. Clench your buttocks and contract your core muscles to help stabilise your spine. Try not to over extend your spine as this can jam the joints into each other. Just rise up enough to give yourself a straight spine.

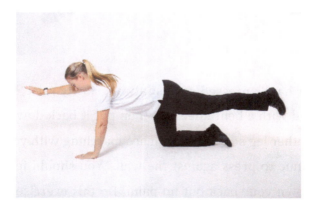

On your hands and knees slowly raise one arm in front of you. If this is easy and you are not wobbling, then try raising the opposite leg as well. Contract your core muscles in this position and hold for 15 seconds. Repeat with the other arm and leg.

How to help eliminate low back pain and achieve long term relief

CHAPTER 11: BALANCING EXERCISES

As we get older or after an injury it is very common for our balance to be affected. First try some balancing exercises holding onto a chair in case you lose your balance. As your confidence increases you can try to let go of the chair.

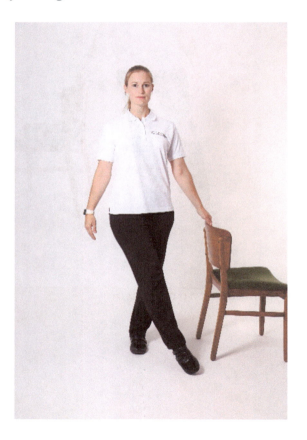

Imagine a clock face on the floor and tap your foot at ten o'clock with or without holding onto the chair.

How to help eliminate low back pain and achieve long term relief

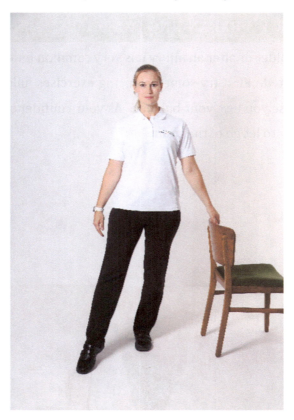

Next, move your foot to two o'clock.

CHAPTER 11: BALANCING EXERCISES

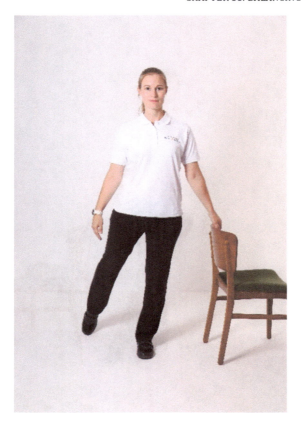

Then move your foot back to around six o'clock. Once this becomes easy you can progress to not holding on to the chair.

Rather than tapping the floor, you can then try lifting your foot just off the floor, which will make things a little harder.

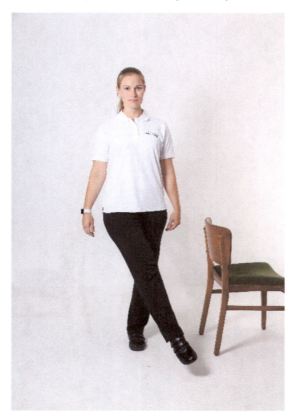

Once this is easy, you can then try doing the exercises with your eyes closed! Just make sure there is something nearby you can grab if you start to lose your balance.

ADVANCED BALANCING EXERCISES

Once you can easily balance with your eyes closed, try doing the same exercises, but this time on a cushion to increase difficulty. Once this becomes easy, you can try closing your eyes on the cushion too.

(See following diagrams).

How to help eliminate low back pain and achieve long term relief

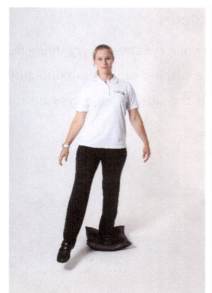
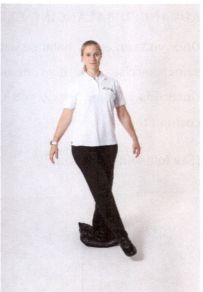
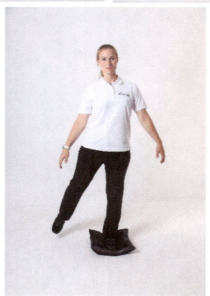

CHAPTER 12: EXERCISES USING A FOAM ROLLER

If you find your muscles feel tight in your legs or back, you could try using a foam roller. This can be quite painful to start with as your muscles will be tight. But if you start by only doing fifteen seconds of rolling on each area and build up each day, it will soon be easier and less painful to do.

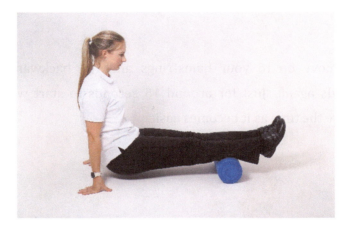

Start with your calf muscles and slowly work your way up your legs. Roll slowly backwards and forwards in the middle of the muscle. Try not to go too near your ankles or knees where the muscle attaches but stay where the muscle is at its biggest.

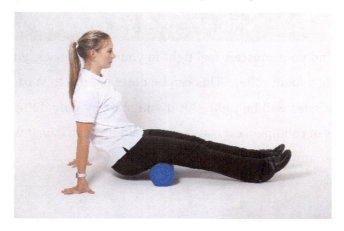

Next, move on to your hamstrings and roll backwards and forwards again. Just for around 15 seconds to start with and increase the time as it becomes easier.

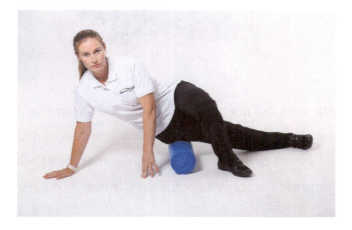

For the side of your leg, called the illio-tibial band (ITB), you need to be on your side, but cross your top leg in front of you to help you balance as you roll up and down the side of your leg. This one tends to be very painful to start with so do just five seconds of rolling to begin with and see how you get on.

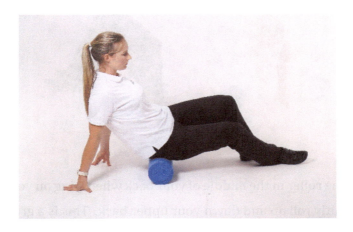

Tilting to your side, sit on the roller to roll on the buttock muscles. This can be a great exercise to help with sciatica and piriformis syndrome. With any back pain, though, these muscles can tighten.

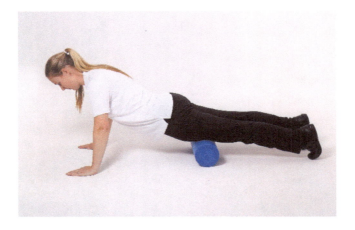

Turn on to your front and roll on the quadriceps muscles.

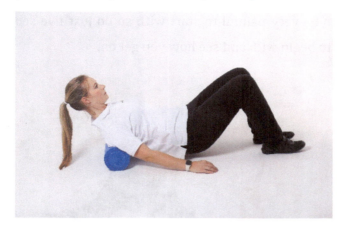

Place the roller in the middle of your back when lying on your back and gently roll up and down your upper back. This is a great way to relieve tension in the back and should feel nice to do.

CHAPTER 13: EXERCISES USING A SQUIDGY BALL

Using a ball like the miracle ball pictured here is a great way to give your muscles a massage, reducing the tension.

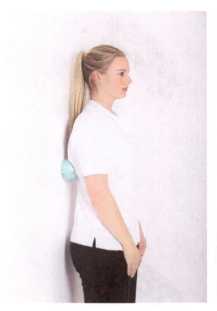
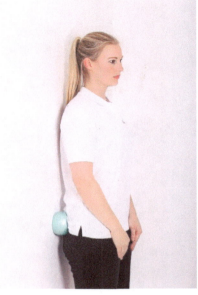

They are quite easy to use against a wall or on the floor. Roll around with them to give yourself a massage.

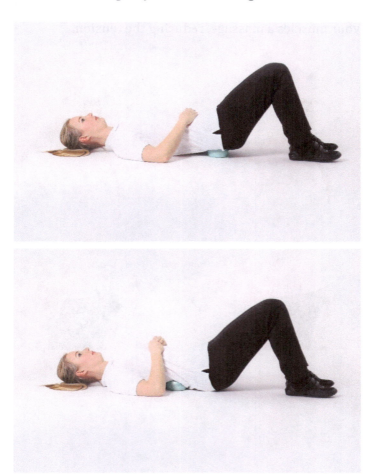

CHAPTER 14: PRODUCTS WHICH MIGHT HELP YOUR BACK PAIN

An ice pack can be used wrapped in a tea towel, for around five to seven minutes at a time, to help take down inflammation and reduce pain, especially if it is a new injury.

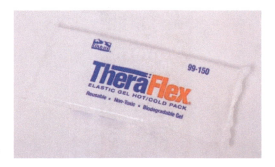

Biofreeze works like an ice pack and is easy to apply to the affected area. It feels all tingly and is a great way of taking your mind off the pain as well as helping with inflammation.

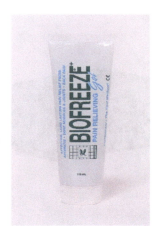

Turmeric taken as a supplement helps with spinal pain and inflammation as well as arthritis.

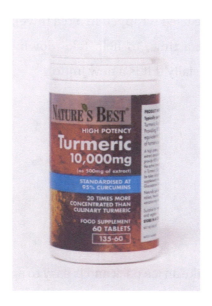

A wedge cushion makes it easier to sit upright in a chair by tilting the pelvis forward.

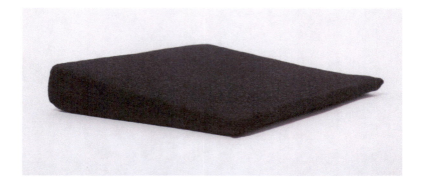

CHAPTER 14: PRODUCTS WHICH MIGHT HELP YOUR BACK PAIN

A lumbar support can be great to have on the sofa to support your back, or in a chair. It makes sure you keep the natural curves in your spine.

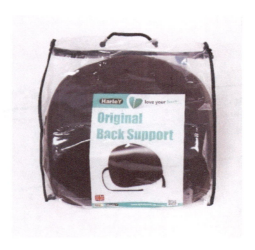

Miracle balls are a great way of massaging the muscles to prevent them from tightening up.

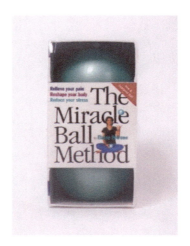

Using a massager is another great way to stop the muscles tightening up too much. This massager is light weight which makes it easy to use.

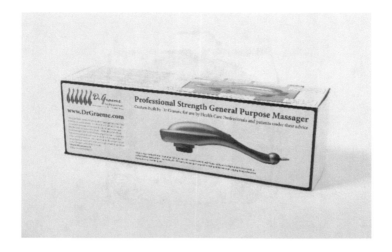

CHAPTER 15: TEN TOP TIPS TO HELP YOUR BACK

TIP 1: BE CAREFUL WHEN YOU FIRST WAKE UP

The back is most vulnerable the first hour after awakening, so make sure you get up slowly and correctly by rolling on your side and getting up from there.

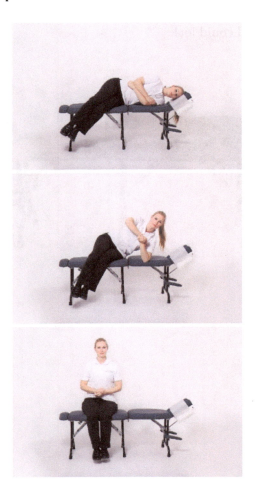

TIP 2: AVOID SLEEPING ON YOUR FRONT

If you sleep on your front your neck has to be twisted to one side and your spine sinks into your stomach and organs; it doesn't have the support it has when you sleep on your side or back. If you have a disc problem lying on your front for short periods can be beneficial, just not all night as this can cause the joints to jam into each other and could lock.

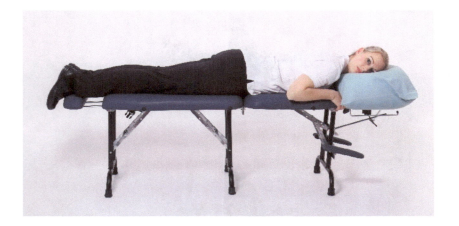

TIP 3: SLEEP WITH A PILLOW UNDER/BETWEEN YOUR LEGS

Using a pillow between your legs when on your side or back really helps to take the pressure off the spine and to put your spine in a great position. This tip won't suit everyone but it is definitely worth a try. A pillow under the knees is preferable to just having your knees bent as it allows your legs to fully relax.

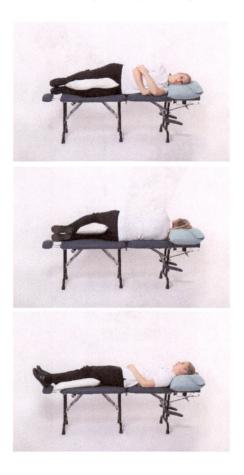

TIP 4: AVOID LOTS OF BENDING

Bending from the back or having bad posture puts extra pressure on the spine. Think about how you do daily activities like unloading a dishwasher or getting out of a chair. Small changes can make a big difference to your back.

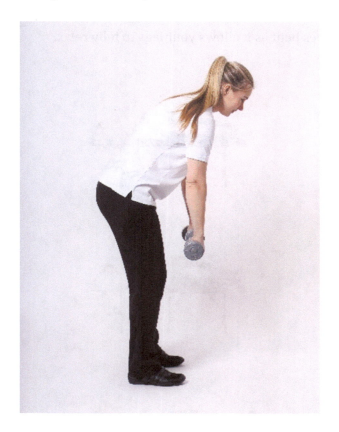

TIP 5: HOLD YOUR PHONE UP

Look at the difference in your posture if you hold your phone up – the pressure on your spine is dramatically reduced.

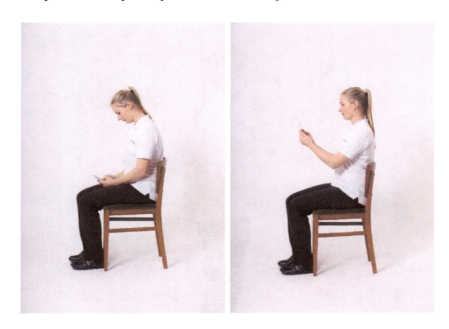

TIP 6: WATCH YOUR POSTURE WHEN STANDING

Every now and then, put your thumbs up and your arms back to help stretch your shoulders back.

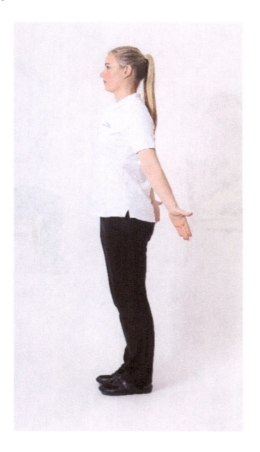

TIP 7: WALK TALL

Imagine being pulled up by your head and lift your sternum to take the pressure off your low back.

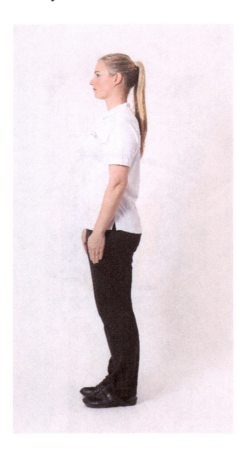

How to help eliminate low back pain and achieve long term relief

TIP 8: WEAR WELL-FITTING SHOES

Best foot forward...make sure your shoes fit well. If you have flat feet, look into orthotics to help distribute the pressure through your feet properly.

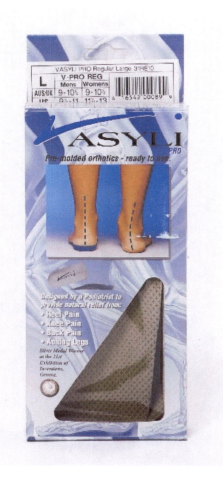

TIP 9: GO FOR A WALK

Walking is fantastic exercise and great for the spine. Make sure you swing your arms as you walk.

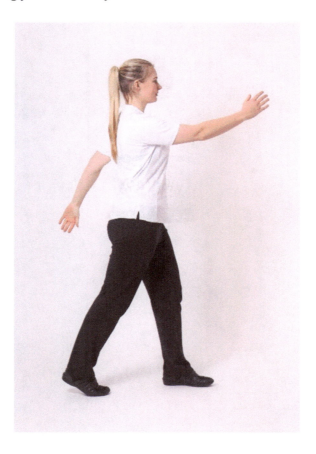

TIP 10: KEEP HYDRATED

Make sure you drink lots of water. This will help your muscles stay healthy and help to prevent them going into spasm.

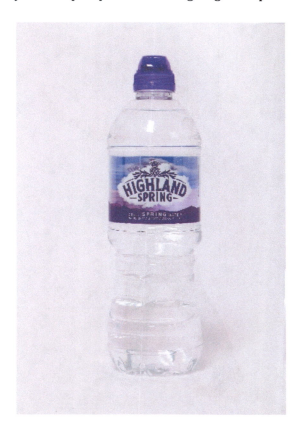

AND FINALLY...

I hope you find this book helpful. As you can see there is no single exercise that will help everyone but, by trying lots of different exercises and listening to your body, you should be able to find out what suits you best and what can help relieve your pain.

The main thing is not to ignore pain, but to find out what is going on and then use treatment, along with exercises to help your pain and prevent it returning.

Back pain is usually caused by a mixture of things, both physical and mental. Posture has a part to play along with bending or lifting.

I hope this book provides you with useful information about the anatomy of the spine, so you can understand where your pain is coming from and can be more aware of how it can be aggravated.

Throughout life, staying active is extremely important, so if pain is preventing you from doing this, you must seek help.

I wish you all the best with your healing journey.

Louise

REFERENCES

Ammendolia C., Côté P., Southerst D., Schneider M., Budgell B., Bombardier C., Hawker G., Rampersaud Y.R. (2018). 'Comprehensive non-surgical treatment versus self-directed care to improve walking ability in lumbar spinal stenosis: A randomized trial.' *Archives of Physical Medicine and Rehabilitation.*

Butler, D.S. (2000) *The Sensitive Nervous System* Noigroup Publications, Australia.

Campbell, P., Bishop, A., Dunn, K.M., Main, C.J., Thomas, E., and Foster, N.E.. (2013) 'Conceptual overlap of psychological constructs in low back pain'. *Pain.* 154: 1783-1791.

Cherkin D.C., Sherman K.J., Balderson B.H., Cook A.J., Anderson M.L., Hawkes R.J., Hansen K.E., and Turner J.A..(2016). 'Effect of mindfulness-based stress reduction vs cognitive behavioral therapy or usual care on back pain and functional limitations in adults with chronic low back pain: a randomized clinical trial.' JAMA. 315(12):1240-1249.

Dagenais S., Gay R.E., Tricco A.C., Freeman M.D., and Mayer J.M.. (2010) 'NASS Contemporary Concepts in Spine Care: spinal manipulation therapy for acute low back pain.' Vol 10, (10); 918-940.

Elrod, H., (2013) The Miracle Morning *Hal Elrod International Inc.*

Foster, N.E., Anema, J.R., Cherkin, D., Chou, R., Cohen, S.P., Gross, D.P., Ferreira, P.H., Fritz,J.M., Koes, B.W., Peul, W., Turner,J.A., and Maher C.G., on behalf of the Lancet Low Back Pain Series Working Group (2018) 'Prevention and treatment of low back pain: evidence, challenges, and promising directions'. *The Lancet*, Vol. 391, No. 10137.

Froud, R., Patterson, S., Eldridge, S., Seale C., Pincus T., Rajendran D., Fossum C., and Underwood M., (2014) 'A systematic review and meta-synthesis of the impact of low back pain on people's lives'. *BMC Musculoskeletal Disorders* 15: 50.

Gifford, L.S., (1998) 'Pain, the tissues and the nervous system'. *Physiotherapy* 84:27-33.

Hartvigsen, J., Hancock, M.J., Kongsted, A., Louw, Q., Ferreira, M.L., Genevay,S., Hoy, D., Karppinen, J., Pransky, G., Sieper, J., Smeets, R. J., and Underwood M., on behalf of the Lancet Low Back Pain Series Working Group (2018) 'What low back pain is and why we need to pay attention'. *The Lancet*, Vol. 391, No. 10137.

Hoy, D., Bain, C., Williams, G., March L., Brooks P., Blyth F., Woolf A., Vos T., and Buchbinder R. (2012) 'A systematic review of the global prevalence of low back pain'. *Arthritis and Rheumatism.* Vol. 64: 2028–2037.

Lewis,R.A., Williams, N.H., Sutton, A.J. Burton,K., Ud Din, N., Matar,H.E., Hendry,M., Phillips,C.J., Nafees, S., Fitzsimmons, D., Rickard,I. and Wilkinson, C. (2015).' Comparative clinical effectiveness of management strategies for sciatica: systematic review and network meta-analyses.' *The Spine Journal.* Vol. 15, (6);1461–1477.

McKenzie, R. (2011) *Treat Your Own Back* Spinal Publications Ltd. New Zealand.

McGill, S. (2002) Low Back Disorders Evidence-Based Prevention and Rehabilitation. Human Kinetics. Champaign, IL.

Nachemson A. (1966) 'The Load on Lumbar Disks in Different Positions of the Body.' *Clin Rel Res,* 45:107.

Petersen, T., Larsen, K., Nordsteen, J., Olsen, S., Fournier, G., and Jacobsen, S., (2011). 'The McKenzie method compared with manipulation when used adjunctive to information and advice in low back pain patients presenting with centralization or peripheralization: a randomized controlled trial'. Spine: Vol. 36 (24) 1999–2010

Turner, J.A., Anderson M.L., Balderson, B.H., Cook, A.J., Sherman, K.J., Cherkin, D.C., (2016) 'Mindfulness-based stress reduction and cognitive-behavioural therapy for chronic low back pain: similar effects on mindfulness, catastrophizing, self-efficacy, and acceptance in randomized controlled trial.' *Pain*. 157 (11) 2434-2444.

http://www.guy-declerck.com/en/lumbar-intervertebral-disc-biomechanical-function